FATTY LIVER AND CIRRHOSIS DIET COOKBOOK FOR NEWLY DIAGNOSED

MEY W SMITH

TABLE OF CONTENTS

3 | FATTY LIVER AND CIRRHOSIS DIET COOKBOOK FOR NEWLY DIAGNOSED

Introduction

A fatty liver and cirrhosis diet cookbook is a resource designed to help individuals manage and mitigate the effects of liver conditions through proper nutrition. Fatty liver disease is characterized by the accumulation of fat in liver cells, while cirrhosis is a more advanced stage of liver damage where healthy tissue is replaced by scar tissue. Both conditions can have various causes, symptoms, and preventive measures.

Fatty Liver Disease

Types:
1. Non-Alcoholic Fatty Liver Disease (NAFLD):- Occurs without excessive alcohol consumption and is often associated with obesity, diabetes, or metabolic syndrome.
2. -Alcoholic Fatty Liver Disease (AFLD):- Results from chronic alcohol consumption, leading to fat accumulation in the liver.

Causes

- -Poor Diet:- High intake of refined carbohydrates, sugar, and saturated fats.
- -Obesity:- Excess body weight, especially abdominal fat, increases the risk.

- -Insulin Resistance:- A condition where cells don't respond effectively to insulin, often linked to type 2 diabetes.
- -Genetics:- Some genetic factors may predispose individuals to fatty liver disease.

Symptoms

- -Fatigue:- Feeling tired and weak.
- -Abdominal Discomfort:- Pain or discomfort in the upper right abdomen.
- -Enlarged Liver:- Detected during a physical examination or imaging tests.
- -Elevated Liver Enzymes:- Abnormal liver function tests.

Preventive Measures

1. -Healthy Diet:- Emphasize fruits, vegetables, whole grains, and lean proteins.
2. -Regular Exercise:- Helps manage weight and improve insulin sensitivity.
3. -Limit Alcohol Intake:- For those with NAFLD, avoiding alcohol is crucial.
4. -Weight Management:- Maintain a healthy weight through diet and exercise.
5. -Control Blood Sugar:- Manage diabetes through medication, diet, and lifestyle changes.

Cirrhosis

Types:

1. -Compensated Cirrhosis:- Early stage with liver damage but still functioning adequately.

2. -Decompensated Cirrhosis:- Advanced stage where the liver can no longer function properly.

Causes

- -Long-term Alcohol Abuse:- A leading cause of cirrhosis.
- -Chronic Viral Hepatitis:- Hepatitis B and C infections can lead to cirrhosis.
- -Non-Alcoholic Steatohepatitis (NASH):- Severe form of NAFLD progressing to cirrhosis.
- -Autoimmune Diseases:- Conditions where the immune system attacks liver cells.

Symptoms

- -Fatigue and Weakness:- Persistent tiredness.
- -Easy Bruising:- Due to decreased production of blood-clotting proteins.
- -Swelling:- Fluid retention leading to edema, especially in the legs and abdomen.

- -Confusion:- Hepatic encephalopathy can cause cognitive impairment.

Preventive Measures

1. -Avoid Alcohol:- For individuals with alcohol-related cirrhosis.
2. -Vaccinations:- Immunization against hepatitis A and B.
3. -Regular Monitoring:- Periodic liver function tests and imaging.
4. -Manage Complications:- Treat and manage complications promptly.
5. -Healthy Lifestyle:- Proper diet, exercise, and stress management.

Chapter 1

Fatty Liver & Cirrhosis Diet Cookbook

Purpose:
- -Tailored Recipes:- Designed to support liver health by incorporating nutrient-rich, liver-friendly ingredients.
- -Balanced Nutrition:- Focus on essential nutrients while minimizing saturated fats, sugar, and processed foods.

Cookbook Content:
1. -Liver-Boosting Recipes:- Featuring foods rich in antioxidants, vitamins, and minerals.
2. -Low-Fat Options:- Emphasizing lean proteins and healthy fats.
3. -Portion Control:- Encouraging mindful eating to manage weight.
4. -Meal Planning:- Structured plans to ensure balanced and varied nutrition.

Practical Tips:
- -Hydration:- Adequate water intake is crucial for liver function.
- -Herbs and Spices:- Incorporating herbs like turmeric known for anti-inflammatory properties.

- -Limiting Salt:- Helps manage fluid retention common in liver conditions.

A Fatty Liver & Cirrhosis Diet Cookbook serves as a valuable tool in managing these liver conditions by promoting a balanced and liver-friendly diet. It complements other preventive measures, such as regular exercise, weight management, and medical interventions. Always consult with healthcare professionals for personalized advice and treatment plans.

Chapter 2

What to eat

A Fatty Liver & Cirrhosis Diet Cookbook is a crucial resource for individuals managing these liver conditions, offering guidance on foods to include and avoid to promote liver health. The emphasis is on supporting liver function, minimizing inflammation, and preventing further damage.

Foods to Include

1. -Fruits and Vegetables:-
   - -Berries:- Rich in antioxidants that combat inflammation.
   - -Leafy Greens:- Spinach, kale, and other greens provide essential vitamins and minerals.
   - -Cruciferous Vegetables:- Broccoli, cauliflower, and Brussels sprouts support detoxification.

2. -Whole Grains:-
   - -Quinoa, Brown Rice, Oats:- High in fiber, aiding digestion and promoting a feeling of fullness.

3. -Lean Proteins:-
   - -Chicken, Turkey, Fish:- Excellent sources of protein with lower fat content.
   - -Plant-Based Proteins:- Tofu, legumes, and beans provide alternative protein sources.

4. -Healthy Fats:-
   - -Avocado:- Contains monounsaturated fats, beneficial for heart health.
   - -Nuts and Seeds:- Almonds, walnuts, flaxseeds offer omega-3 fatty acids.

5. -Dairy or Alternatives:-
   - -Low-Fat Dairy:- Milk, yogurt, and cheese in moderation for calcium and protein.
   - -Plant-Based Alternatives:- Almond or soy milk for those with lactose intolerance.

6. -Herbs and Spices:-
   - -Turmeric:- Known for its anti-inflammatory properties.
   - -Garlic:- Supports liver function and has potential anti-inflammatory effects.

7. -Hydration:-
   - -Water:- Essential for overall health and aids in flushing toxins from the body.

Foods to Limit or Avoid

1. -Saturated and Trans Fats:-
   - -Processed Foods:- Fast food, fried items, and packaged snacks often contain unhealthy fats.
   - -Red Meat:- Limit intake and opt for lean cuts.

13 | FATTY LIVER AND CIRRHOSIS DIET COOKBOOK FOR NEWLY DIAGNOSED

2. -Added Sugars:-

   - -Sweets and Sugary Beverages:- Cookies, cakes, soda contribute to fat accumulation in the liver.

   - -High-Fructose Corn Syrup:- Found in many processed foods and sugary drinks.

3. -Salt:-

   - -Processed and Canned Foods:- High in sodium, contributing to fluid retention.

   - -Table Salt:- Limit added salt during cooking and at the table.

4. -Alcohol:-

   - -Complete Abstinence:- For individuals with liver conditions, alcohol can exacerbate damage.

5. -Refined Carbohydrates:-

   - -White Bread, Pasta, and Rice:- Opt for whole grains for better fiber content.

6. -High-Protein Diets:-

   - -Moderation is Key:- Excessive protein can strain the liver, so balance intake.

7. -Unnecessary Supplements:-

- -Consult with Healthcare Providers:- Avoid self-prescribing supplements, as some may interact with medications or affect the liver.

Practical Tips for a Fatty Liver & Cirrhosis Diet

1. -Portion Control:- Manage calorie intake to maintain a healthy weight.
2. -Meal Timing:- Regular, balanced meals and snacks throughout the day.
3. -Moderate Cooking Methods:- Choose baking, steaming, or grilling over frying.
4. -Mindful Eating:- Pay attention to hunger and fullness cues.

A well-structured Fatty Liver & Cirrhosis Diet Cookbook provides not only a list of foods but also practical recipes and meal plans that incorporate these guidelines. It promotes a balanced and varied diet to ensure individuals receive essential nutrients while minimizing factors that could worsen liver conditions. As always, it's essential for individuals with liver conditions to consult with healthcare professionals for personalized dietary recommendations based on their specific health needs and medical history.

Following a Fatty Liver & Cirrhosis Diet Cookbook can provide several core benefits for individuals managing these liver conditions. The cookbook is designed to offer guidance on nutrition, promote liver health, and assist in preventing further damage.

Here are key benefits:

1. -Liver Support:-

 - -Balanced Nutrition:- The cookbook emphasizes a well-balanced diet rich in essential nutrients, supporting overall liver function.

 - -Anti-Inflammatory Foods:- Incorporating foods with anti-inflammatory properties, such as fruits, vegetables, and herbs, can help reduce liver inflammation.

2. -Weight Management:-

 - -Portion Control:- The cookbook often encourages mindful eating and portion control, which is crucial for managing body weight – a key factor in liver health.

 - -Healthy Fats:- Emphasizing the consumption of healthy fats can contribute to weight management by providing satiety without contributing to excessive calorie intake.

3. -Minimization of Liver Fat Accumulation:-

 - -Low-Fat Options:- The cookbook promotes recipes with lower fat content, assisting in preventing further fat accumulation in the liver.

- -Avoidance of Unhealthy Fats:- By steering individuals away from saturated and trans fats, the cookbook helps reduce the burden on the liver.

4. -Blood Sugar Control:-
   - -Complex Carbohydrates:- Encouraging the consumption of whole grains helps stabilize blood sugar levels, benefiting individuals with conditions like non-alcoholic fatty liver disease (NAFLD) linked to insulin resistance.

5. -Heart Health:-
   - -Omega-3 Fatty Acids:- Including sources of omega-3s, such as fish and nuts, promotes cardiovascular health, crucial for individuals with liver conditions often associated with heart-related complications.

6. -Reduced Sodium Intake:-
   - -Limiting Fluid Retention:- The cookbook advises on minimizing salt intake, which helps manage fluid retention, a common issue in liver conditions like cirrhosis.

7. -Improved Digestion:-
   - -High-Fiber Foods:- Whole grains, fruits, and vegetables included in the cookbook provide dietary fiber, promoting healthy digestion and preventing constipation.

8. -Nutrient-Rich Options:-

- -Vitamins and Minerals:- The cookbook emphasizes foods rich in essential vitamins and minerals, supporting overall health and addressing potential deficiencies associated with liver conditions.

9. -Hydration:-

- -Water Emphasis:- Adequate hydration is crucial for liver function and overall health. The cookbook likely encourages sufficient water intake.

10. -Psychological Well-being:-

- -Structured Meal Plans:- Having a structured approach to meals and snacks can contribute to a sense of control and well-being, reducing stress associated with managing dietary restrictions.

11. -Education and Empowerment:-

- -Understanding Dietary Impact:- The cookbook educates individuals on how specific foods can impact liver health, empowering them to make informed choices.

12. -Preventive Measures:-

- -Alcohol Abstinence:- For those with alcohol-related liver conditions, the cookbook reinforces the importance of complete abstinence from alcohol, a crucial preventive measure.

13. -Practical Guidance:-

- -Recipes and Meal Plans:- Providing practical recipes and meal plans makes it easier for individuals to follow the dietary recommendations consistently.

While a Fatty Liver & Cirrhosis Diet Cookbook offers valuable guidance, it's essential for individuals to use it in conjunction with medical advice. Consulting with healthcare professionals ensures that the dietary recommendations align with individual health needs, medical history, and specific liver conditions.

Chapter 3

How to follow

Following a Fatty Liver & Cirrhosis Diet Cookbook involves a combination of understanding the dietary guidelines provided and incorporating them into your daily life. Here's a step-by-step guide on how to effectively follow such a diet cookbook:

1. -Acquire the Cookbook:-
   - Purchase or access a Fatty Liver & Cirrhosis Diet Cookbook that aligns with your dietary preferences and needs.

2. -Read and Understand Guidelines:-
   - Thoroughly read the introduction and guidelines provided in the cookbook. Understand the principles behind the recommended foods and restrictions.

3. -Consult with Healthcare Professionals:-
   - Before making significant dietary changes, consult with your healthcare team, including a hepatologist or nutritionist, to ensure the recommendations suit your specific health condition.

4. -Create a Meal Plan:-

 - Use the cookbook's meal plans and recipes to create a structured daily or weekly meal plan. Ensure it includes a variety of nutrient-dense foods.

5. -Grocery Shopping:-

 - Compile a grocery list based on the recipes and meal plan. Prioritize fresh fruits, vegetables, lean proteins, whole grains, and other recommended items.

6. -Meal Preparation:-

 - Set aside dedicated time for meal preparation. Follow recipes provided in the cookbook, paying attention to portion sizes and cooking methods (e.g., baking, steaming).

7. -Mindful Eating:-

 - Practice mindful eating by savoring each bite and paying attention to hunger and fullness cues. Avoid distractions like phones or TV during meals.

8. -Hydration:-

 - Emphasize adequate water intake. Water is essential for overall health and supports liver function.

9. -Portion Control:-

- Be mindful of portion sizes. Overeating, even with healthy foods, can contribute to excess calorie intake.

10. -Regular Eating Schedule:-
  - Stick to a regular eating schedule with balanced meals and snacks. Avoid long periods of fasting.

11. -Avoid Restricted Foods:-
  - Strictly adhere to the guidelines regarding foods to avoid, such as those high in saturated fats, added sugars, and excessive sodium.

12. -Alcohol Abstinence:-
  - If the cookbook recommends alcohol abstinence, adhere to this restriction completely.

13. -Monitor and Adjust:-
  - Keep track of how your body responds to the dietary changes. Note any improvements in energy levels, digestion, or other relevant aspects.

14. -Regular Check-ins with Healthcare Team:-
  - Schedule regular check-ins with your healthcare team to discuss progress, address concerns, and make any necessary adjustments to the diet plan.

15. -Incorporate Physical Activity:-

- Combine the dietary changes with regular physical activity, as approved by your healthcare provider. Exercise supports overall health and can aid in weight management.

16. -Educate Yourself:-
- Continuously educate yourself about the impact of specific foods on liver health. Stay informed about new recipes and research related to Fatty Liver & Cirrhosis diets.

17. -Seek Support:-
- If possible, join support groups or communities with individuals facing similar dietary challenges. Sharing experiences and tips can provide valuable insights.

18. -Stay Positive and Patient:-
- Understand that changes in health and well-being may take time. Stay positive, be patient with the process, and celebrate small victories along the way.

19. -Reassess and Adjust as Needed:-
- Periodically reassess your diet plan in consultation with your healthcare team. Adjustments may be necessary based on your health status and progress.

20. -Long-Term Commitment:-

- Recognize that following a Fatty Liver & Cirrhosis Diet is often a long-term commitment. Make it a sustainable part of your lifestyle for lasting health benefits.

Remember, individual dietary needs may vary, and personalization is crucial. Always consult with healthcare professionals before making significant changes to your diet, especially if you have underlying health conditions.

Shopping ingredients

Certainly! When shopping for a Fatty Liver & Cirrhosis Diet Cookbook, focus on incorporating nutrient-dense, liver-friendly ingredients. Here's a list of 20 healthy shopping ingredients for such a diet:

Fruits and Vegetables:
1. -Berries:- Blueberries, strawberries, raspberries - rich in antioxidants.
2. -Leafy Greens:- Spinach, kale, Swiss chard - high in vitamins and minerals.
3. -Citrus Fruits:- Oranges, grapefruits, lemons - a good source of vitamin C.
4. -Avocado:- Contains monounsaturated fats and supports liver health.

Whole Grains:
5. -Quinoa:- A complete protein with high fiber content.
6. -Brown Rice:- Provides complex carbohydrates and fiber.

7. -Oats:- High in soluble fiber, beneficial for digestion.

Lean Proteins:
8. -Chicken Breast:- Lean source of protein.
9. -Turkey:- Low-fat alternative to red meat.
10. -Fatty Fish:- Salmon, mackerel, trout - rich in omega-3 fatty acids.

Plant-Based Proteins:
11. -Tofu:- A versatile, plant-based protein.
12. -Legumes:- Lentils, chickpeas, black beans - high in fiber and protein.
13. -Quinoa:- A complete protein with high fiber content.

Healthy Fats:
14. -Olive Oil:- Contains monounsaturated fats and antioxidants.
15. -Nuts and Seeds:- Almonds, walnuts, flaxseeds - provide omega-3 fatty acids.
16. -Chia Seeds:- High in fiber, omega-3s, and antioxidants.

Dairy or Alternatives:
17. -Low-Fat Yogurt:- A good source of protein and calcium.
18. -Almond Milk:- A plant-based alternative for those with lactose intolerance.

Herbs and Spices:

19. -Turmeric:- Known for its anti-inflammatory properties.
20. -Garlic:- Supports liver function and adds flavor to dishes.

Bonus Tips:
- -Fresh Herbs:- Parsley, cilantro, basil - add flavor without added salt.
- -Colorful Vegetables:- Aim for a variety of colors for a diverse range of nutrients.
- -Eggs:- A good source of protein, but consult with healthcare professionals regarding individual dietary needs.
- -Low-Sodium Broth:- Use for cooking and flavoring without excessive salt.
- -Green Tea:- Known for antioxidants and potential liver benefits.

When shopping, opt for fresh, whole foods and minimize processed items. Always read labels for hidden sugars, saturated fats, and excessive sodium. Additionally, consider consulting with a healthcare professional or nutritionist for personalized advice based on individual health needs and the specific stage of Fatty Liver or Cirrhosis.

Chapter 4

7 Day Meal Plan

Certainly, here's a sample 7-day Fatty Liver & Cirrhosis Diet Cookbook plan. Please note that individual dietary needs may vary, and it's crucial to consult with healthcare professionals for personalized advice.

Day 1:
-Breakfast:-
- Oatmeal with sliced strawberries and a sprinkle of chia seeds.
- Green tea.

-Lunch:-
- Grilled chicken breast with quinoa and steamed broccoli.
- Mixed green salad with olive oil dressing.

-Dinner:-
- Baked salmon with lemon and herbs.
- Sweet potato wedges.
- Sautéed spinach with garlic.

Day 2:
-Breakfast:-
- Whole grain toast with avocado slices.
- Greek yogurt with blueberries.

-Lunch:-
- Lentil and vegetable soup.
- Quinoa salad with cherry tomatoes and cucumber.

-Dinner:-
- Stir-fried tofu with colorful bell peppers and snap peas.
- Brown rice.

Day 3:
-Breakfast:-
- Scrambled eggs with sautéed spinach.
- Orange slices.

-Lunch:-
- Turkey and vegetable wrap with whole wheat tortilla.
- Mixed fruit salad.

-Dinner:-
- Grilled mackerel with a side of roasted Brussels sprouts.
- Quinoa pilaf.

Day 4:
-Breakfast:-
- Smoothie with kale, banana, and almond milk.
- Handful of almonds.

-Lunch:-

- Chickpea salad with cherry tomatoes, cucumber, and feta.

- Whole grain crackers.

-Dinner:-

- Baked chicken with rosemary and lemon.

- Steamed asparagus and carrots.

Day 5:

-Breakfast:-

- Overnight oats with sliced peaches and a drizzle of honey.

- Green tea.

-Lunch:-

- Caprese salad with tomatoes, mozzarella, and fresh basil.

- Grilled chicken strips.

-Dinner:-

- Stir-fried shrimp with broccoli and snow peas.

- Quinoa.

Day 6:

-Breakfast:-

- Whole grain bagel with smoked salmon and cream cheese.

- Mixed berries.

-Lunch:-

- Brown rice bowl with black beans, corn, and avocado.

- Side of salsa.

-Dinner:-
- Oven-roasted cod with lemon and dill.
- Sweet potato mash.
Day 7:
-Breakfast:-
- Spinach and feta omelet.
- Fresh orange slices.

-Lunch:-
- Turkey and vegetable stir-fry with quinoa.
- Mixed green salad with balsamic vinaigrette.

-Dinner:-
- Grilled vegetable skewers with tofu.
- Wild rice pilaf.

Feel free to repeat or modify this plan based on personal preferences, and remember to stay hydrated with water throughout the day. This sample plan provides a variety of nutrient-dense foods to support liver health while offering delicious and satisfying meals. Adjust portion sizes based on individual needs and consult with healthcare professionals for any necessary modifications.

Chapter 5

Breakfast

1. Oatmeal with Berries

-Ingredients:-
- 1/2 cup rolled oats
- 1 cup water or almond milk
- 1/2 cup mixed berries (blueberries, strawberries)
- 1 tablespoon chia seeds

-Preparation:-
1. In a saucepan, bring water or almond milk to a boil.
2. Add rolled oats and cook on medium heat for 5-7 minutes, stirring occasionally.
3. Once cooked, top with mixed berries and chia seeds.

-Nutritional Value:-
- Calories: ~300
- Fiber: ~8g
- Protein: ~10g
- Cooking Time: 10 minutes

2. Avocado Toast with Poached Egg

-Ingredients:-
- 1 slice whole grain bread

- 1/2 ripe avocado
- 1 poached egg
- Salt and pepper to taste

-Preparation:-
1. Toast the whole grain bread.
2. Mash the avocado and spread it on the toast.
3. Top with a poached egg. Season with salt and pepper.

-Nutritional Value:-
- Calories: ~250
- Fiber: ~7g
- Protein: ~12g
- Cooking Time: 15 minutes

3. Greek Yogurt Parfait

-Ingredients:-
- 1 cup plain Greek yogurt
- 1/2 cup granola (low-sugar)
- 1/2 cup mixed berries
- 1 tablespoon honey

-Preparation:-
1. In a glass or bowl, layer Greek yogurt, granola, and mixed berries.
2. Drizzle honey on top.

-Nutritional Value:-
- Calories: ~300
- Protein: ~20g
- Fiber: ~5g
- Cooking Time: 5 minutes

4. Quinoa Breakfast Bowl

-Ingredients:-
- 1/2 cup cooked quinoa
- 1/4 cup almond milk
- 1/2 banana, sliced
- 1 tablespoon sliced almonds
- Cinnamon to taste

-Preparation:-
1. Mix cooked quinoa with almond milk.
2. Top with banana slices, sliced almonds, and a sprinkle of cinnamon.

-Nutritional Value:-
- Calories: ~250
- Protein: ~8g
- Fiber: ~5g
- Cooking Time: 10 minutes

5. Smoothie Bowl

-Ingredients:-
- 1 cup spinach
- 1/2 frozen banana
- 1/2 cup frozen berries
- 1/2 cup almond milk
- 1 tablespoon chia seeds

-Preparation:-
1. Blend spinach, banana, berries, and almond milk until smooth.
2. Pour into a bowl and top with chia seeds.

-Nutritional Value:-
- Calories: ~200
- Protein: ~5g
- Fiber: ~8g
- Cooking Time: 5 minutes

6. Chia Seed Pudding

-Ingredients:-
- 2 tablespoons chia seeds
- 1/2 cup almond milk
- 1/2 teaspoon vanilla extract
- Sliced kiwi for topping

-Preparation:-

1. Mix chia seeds, almond milk, and vanilla extract in a bowl.
2. Refrigerate for at least 2 hours or overnight.
3. Top with sliced kiwi before serving.

-Nutritional Value:-
- Calories: ~150
- Protein: ~5g
- Fiber: ~8g
- Cooking Time: 2 hours (mostly refrigeration time)

7. Egg White Veggie Scramble

-Ingredients:-
- 3 egg whites
- 1/4 cup diced bell peppers
- 1/4 cup diced tomatoes
- Spinach leaves
- Salt and pepper to taste

-Preparation:-
1. Whisk egg whites and pour into a heated, non-stick skillet.
2. Add bell peppers, tomatoes, and spinach. Scramble until cooked.
3. Season with salt and pepper.

-Nutritional Value:-

- Calories: ~150
- Protein: ~20g
- Cooking Time: 10 minutes

8. Chickpea and Spinach Breakfast Wrap

-Ingredients:-
- 1 whole grain wrap
- 1/2 cup chickpeas (canned, rinsed)
- Handful of spinach leaves
- Sliced cucumber
- Hummus for spreading

-Preparation:-
1. Spread hummus on the wrap.
2. Fill with chickpeas, spinach, and cucumber.
3. Roll up and enjoy.

-Nutritional Value:-
- Calories: ~300
- Protein: ~15g
- Fiber: ~8g
- Cooking Time: 10 minutes

9. Whole Grain Pancakes with Fruit

-Ingredients:-
- 1/2 cup whole grain pancake mix

- 1/3 cup water
- Sliced strawberries and bananas for topping

-Preparation:-
1. Mix pancake mix with water.
2. Cook pancakes on a non-stick skillet.
3. Top with sliced strawberries and bananas.

-Nutritional Value:-
- Calories: ~250
- Protein: ~6g
- Fiber: ~4g
- Cooking Time: 15 minutes

10. Cottage Cheese and Pineapple Bowl

-Ingredients:-
- 1/2 cup low-fat cottage cheese
- 1/2 cup fresh pineapple chunks
- 1 tablespoon shredded coconut

-Preparation:-
1. Mix cottage cheese with pineapple chunks.
2. Top with shredded coconut.

-Nutritional Value:-
- Calories: ~200

- Protein: ~15g
- Cooking Time: 5 minutes

These breakfast recipes are designed to be nutritious and supportive of liver health. Adjust portion sizes based on individual needs and consult with healthcare professionals for any necessary modifications.

Chapter 6

Launch

1. Grilled Chicken and Quinoa Salad

-Ingredients:-
- 4 oz grilled chicken breast, sliced
- 1/2 cup cooked quinoa
- Mixed greens (spinach, arugula)
- Cherry tomatoes, halved
- Cucumber, sliced
- Olive oil and lemon dressing

-Preparation:-
1. Grill chicken breast until fully cooked.
2. Assemble salad with mixed greens, quinoa, cherry tomatoes, and cucumber.
3. Top with grilled chicken slices and drizzle with olive oil and lemon dressing.

-Nutritional Value:-
- Calories: ~400
- Protein: ~30g
- Fiber: ~8g
- Cooking Time: 20 minutes

2. Lentil and Vegetable Soup

-Ingredients:-
- 1 cup cooked lentils
- 1/2 cup diced carrots
- 1/2 cup diced celery
- 1/2 cup diced zucchini
- Low-sodium vegetable broth
- Garlic and onion for flavor
- Fresh herbs (parsley, thyme)

-Preparation:-
1. Sauté garlic and onion in a pot.
2. Add diced vegetables and cook until slightly tender.
3. Pour in vegetable broth and cooked lentils.
4. Simmer until vegetables are fully cooked. Garnish with fresh herbs.

-Nutritional Value:-
- Calories: ~300
- Protein: ~15g
- Fiber: ~12g
- Cooking Time: 30 minutes

3. Salmon and Quinoa Bowl

-Ingredients:-

- 4 oz baked or grilled salmon fillet
- 1/2 cup cooked quinoa
- Steamed broccoli florets
- Sliced bell peppers
- Lemon-tahini dressing

-Preparation:-
1. Bake or grill salmon until fully cooked.
2. Assemble a bowl with quinoa, steamed broccoli, and sliced bell peppers.
3. Top with salmon and drizzle with lemon-tahini dressing.

-Nutritional Value:-
- Calories: ~450
- Protein: ~30g
- Fiber: ~8g
- Cooking Time: 25 minutes

4. Turkey and Veggie Stir-Fry

-Ingredients:-
- 4 oz lean ground turkey
- Mixed stir-fry vegetables (broccoli, bell peppers, snap peas)
- Low-sodium soy sauce
- Garlic and ginger for flavor
- Brown rice

-Preparation:-

1. Cook ground turkey in a skillet until browned.

2. Add mixed vegetables, garlic, and ginger.

3. Stir-fry until vegetables are tender. Serve over brown rice.

-Nutritional Value:-

- Calories: ~350

- Protein: ~25g

- Fiber: ~6g

- Cooking Time: 20 minutes

5. Mackerel and Quinoa Salad

-Ingredients:-

- 4 oz grilled or baked mackerel fillet

- 1/2 cup cooked quinoa

- Arugula and baby spinach mix

- Sliced cucumbers

- Cherry tomatoes, halved

- Balsamic vinaigrette

-Preparation:-

1. Grill or bake mackerel until fully cooked.

2. Combine quinoa, arugula, baby spinach, sliced cucumbers, and cherry tomatoes.

3. Top with mackerel and drizzle with balsamic vinaigrette.

-Nutritional Value:-

- Calories: ~380

- Protein: ~20g
- Fiber: ~7g
- Cooking Time: 25 minutes

6. Chickpea and Vegetable Wrap

-Ingredients:-
- 1 whole grain wrap
- 1/2 cup canned chickpeas, rinsed and mashed
- Sliced tomatoes, cucumbers, and bell peppers
- Hummus for spreading
- Fresh herbs (cilantro, parsley)

-Preparation:-
1. Spread hummus on the wrap.
2. Fill with mashed chickpeas, sliced tomatoes, cucumbers, and bell peppers.
3. Garnish with fresh herbs before rolling up.

-Nutritional Value:-
- Calories: ~320
- Protein: ~15g
- Fiber: ~8g
- Cooking Time: 10 minutes

7. Stir-Fried Tofu with Vegetables

-Ingredients:-

- 1 cup firm tofu, cubed
- Mixed stir-fry vegetables (broccoli, bell peppers, snow peas)
- Low-sodium teriyaki sauce
- Brown rice

-Preparation:-
1. Stir-fry cubed tofu until golden brown.
2. Add mixed vegetables and stir-fry until tender.
3. Pour low-sodium teriyaki sauce and continue cooking.
4. Serve over brown rice.

-Nutritional Value:-
- Calories: ~380
- Protein: ~20g
- Fiber: ~9g
- Cooking Time: 20 minutes

8. Turkey and Quinoa Stuffed Bell Peppers

-Ingredients:-
- Bell peppers, halved
- 1/2 cup cooked quinoa
- 4 oz lean ground turkey
- Diced tomatoes
- Low-sodium tomato sauce
- Italian seasoning

-Preparation:-

1. Preheat the oven. Place halved bell peppers in a baking dish.

2. Cook ground turkey until browned. Mix with cooked quinoa, diced tomatoes, and Italian seasoning.

3. Stuff bell peppers with the turkey and quinoa mixture.

4. Pour low-sodium tomato sauce over the peppers.

5. Bake until peppers are tender.

-Nutritional Value:-
- Calories: ~320
- Protein: ~20g
- Fiber: ~7g
- Cooking Time: 40 minutes

9. Veggie and Hummus Wrap

-Ingredients:-
- 1 whole grain wrap
- Hummus for spreading
- Sliced cucumber, tomatoes, and bell peppers
- Mixed greens (lettuce, spinach)

-Preparation:-

1. Spread hummus on the wrap.

2. Layer with sliced cucumber, tomatoes, bell peppers, and mixed greens.

3. Roll up and enjoy.

45 | FATTY LIVER AND CIRRHOSIS DIET COOKBOOK FOR NEWLY DIAGNOSED

-Nutritional Value:-
- Calories: ~250
- Protein: ~8g
- Fiber: ~6g
- Cooking Time: 10 minutes

10. Spinach and Feta Omelet

-Ingredients:-
- 3 egg whites
- Handful of spinach leaves
- 2 tablespoons crumbled feta cheese
- Diced tomatoes
- Salt and pepper to taste

-Preparation:-
1. Whisk egg whites and pour into a heated, non-stick skillet.
2. Add spinach, feta, and diced tomatoes.
3. Cook until the omelet is set. Season with salt and pepper.

-Nutritional Value:-
- Calories: ~200
- Protein: ~15g
- Cooking Time: 10 minutes

These lunch recipes are designed to be nutritious and supportive of liver health. Adjust portion sizes based on individual needs and consult with healthcare professionals for any necessary modifications.

Chapter 7

Dinner

1. Baked Chicken with Roasted Vegetables

-Ingredients:-
- 4 oz boneless, skinless chicken breast
- Mixed vegetables (bell peppers, zucchini, cherry tomatoes)
- Olive oil, garlic, and herbs for seasoning

-Preparation:-
1. Preheat the oven. Season chicken with olive oil, garlic, and herbs.
2. Place chicken and mixed vegetables on a baking sheet.
3. Bake until chicken is fully cooked and vegetables are tender.

-Nutritional Value:-
- Calories: ~350
- Protein: ~30g
- Fiber: ~8g
- Cooking Time: 30 minutes

2. Salmon with Lemon-Dill Sauce

-Ingredients:-
- 4 oz salmon fillet

- Lemon juice, dill, and garlic for seasoning
- Steamed asparagus spears
-Preparation:-
1. Preheat the oven. Season salmon with lemon juice, dill, and garlic.
2. Bake until salmon flakes easily with a fork.
3. Serve with steamed asparagus.

-Nutritional Value:-
- Calories: ~400
- Protein: ~25g
- Fiber: ~6g
- Cooking Time: 20 minutes

3. Quinoa-Stuffed Bell Peppers

-Ingredients:-
- Bell peppers, halved
- 1/2 cup cooked quinoa
- Black beans, corn, diced tomatoes
- Cumin and chili powder for seasoning

-Preparation:-
1. Preheat the oven. Place halved bell peppers in a baking dish.
2. Mix cooked quinoa with black beans, corn, diced tomatoes, cumin, and chili powder.
3. Stuff bell peppers with the quinoa mixture.

4. Bake until peppers are tender.

-Nutritional Value:-
- Calories: ~300
- Protein: ~15g
- Fiber: ~8g
- Cooking Time: 35 minutes

4. Tofu and Vegetable Stir-Fry

-Ingredients:-
- 1 cup firm tofu, cubed
- Mixed stir-fry vegetables (broccoli, carrots, snap peas)
- Low-sodium soy sauce and ginger for flavor
- Brown rice

-Preparation:-
1. Stir-fry cubed tofu until golden brown.
2. Add mixed vegetables, soy sauce, and ginger.
3. Stir-fry until vegetables are tender. Serve over brown rice.

-Nutritional Value:-
- Calories: ~350
- Protein: ~20g
- Fiber: ~9g
- Cooking Time: 25 minutes

5. Turkey and Spinach Meatballs

-Ingredients:-
- Lean ground turkey
- Chopped spinach
- Garlic, onion, and Italian herbs for flavor
- Whole grain pasta
- Low-sodium tomato sauce

-Preparation:-
1. Mix ground turkey with chopped spinach, garlic, onion, and Italian herbs.
2. Form into meatballs and bake until cooked through.
3. Serve over whole grain pasta with low-sodium tomato sauce.

-Nutritional Value:-
- Calories: ~380
- Protein: ~25g
- Fiber: ~10g
- Cooking Time: 30 minutes

6. -Chickpea and Tomato Salad:-
-Ingredients:-
- Canned chickpeas, drained
- Cherry tomatoes, halved
- Cucumber, diced
- Red onion, thinly sliced

- Fresh parsley and lemon dressing

-Preparation:-
1. Combine chickpeas, cherry tomatoes, cucumber, and red onion.
2. Toss with fresh parsley and lemon dressing.
-Nutritional Value:-
- Calories: ~250
- Protein: ~10g
- Fiber: ~8g
- Cooking Time: 10 minutes

7. Mushroom and Spinach Quiche

-Ingredients:-
- Whole grain pie crust
- Eggs or egg whites
- Mushrooms, sliced
- Fresh spinach leaves
- Low-fat cheese
- Salt and pepper to taste

-Preparation:-
1. Preheat the oven. Line the pie crust with sliced mushrooms and fresh spinach.
2. In a bowl, whisk eggs (or egg whites) and pour over the vegetables.

3. Sprinkle low-fat cheese on top. Season with salt and pepper.
4. Bake until the quiche is set.

-Nutritional Value:-
- Calories: ~300
- Protein: ~15g
- Fiber: ~6g
- Cooking Time: 40 minutes

8. Stuffed Acorn Squash

-Ingredients:-
- Acorn squash, halved
- Quinoa, black beans, corn, diced tomatoes
- Cumin and chili powder for seasoning

-Preparation:-
1. Preheat the oven. Place acorn squash halves in a baking dish.
2. Mix cooked quinoa with black beans, corn, diced tomatoes, cumin, and chili powder.
3. Stuff acorn squash with the quinoa mixture.
4. Bake until squash is tender.

-Nutritional Value:-
- Calories: ~350
- Protein: ~12g

- Fiber: ~10g
- Cooking Time: 45 minutes

9. Eggplant and Tomato Bake

-Ingredients:-
- Eggplant, sliced
- Sliced tomatoes
- Garlic, thyme, and olive oil for seasoning
- Low-fat mozzarella cheese
-Preparation:-
1. Preheat the oven. Arrange sliced eggplant and tomatoes in a baking dish.
2. Drizzle with olive oil and season with garlic and thyme.
3. Top with low-fat mozzarella cheese.
4. Bake until eggplant is tender and cheese is melted.

-Nutritional Value:-
- Calories: ~280
- Protein: ~15g
- Fiber: ~10g
- Cooking Time: 30 minutes

10. Grilled Shrimp and Quinoa Bowl

-Ingredients:-
- Grilled shrimp
- 1/2 cup cooked quinoa

- Sliced bell peppers and red onion
- Fresh cilantro and lime dressing

-Preparation:-
1. Grill shrimp until cooked.
2. Assemble a bowl with cooked quinoa, sliced bell peppers, red onion, and grilled shrimp.
3. Garnish with fresh cilantro and drizzle with lime dressing.

-Nutritional Value:-
- Calories: ~350
- Protein: ~20g
- Fiber: ~7g
- Cooking Time: 20 minutes

These dinner recipes are designed to be nutritious and supportive of liver health. Adjust portion sizes based on individual needs and consult with healthcare professionals for any necessary modifications.

Chapter 8

Snack

1. Greek Yogurt and Berry Parfait

-Ingredients:-
- 1 cup plain Greek yogurt
- Mixed berries (blueberries, strawberries)
- 2 tablespoons granola (low-sugar)
- 1 tablespoon honey

-Preparation:-
1. In a glass or bowl, layer Greek yogurt, mixed berries, and granola.
2. Drizzle honey on top.

-Nutritional Value:-
- Calories: ~200
- Protein: ~15g
- Fiber: ~4g
- Cooking Time: 5 minutes

2. Avocado and Tomato Salsa

-Ingredients:-
- 1 ripe avocado, diced
- Cherry tomatoes, diced

- Red onion, finely chopped
- Fresh cilantro, chopped
- Lime juice
- Whole grain crackers for serving

-Preparation:-
1. In a bowl, combine diced avocado, tomatoes, red onion, and cilantro.
2. Squeeze lime juice over the mixture.
3. Serve with whole grain crackers.

-Nutritional Value:-
- Calories: ~180
- Protein: ~3g
- Fiber: ~6g
- Cooking Time: 10 minutes

3. Hummus and Veggie Sticks

-Ingredients:-
- Hummus (store-bought or homemade)
- Carrot sticks, cucumber slices, bell pepper strips

-Preparation:-
1. Cut vegetables into sticks or slices.
2. Serve with hummus for dipping.

-Nutritional Value:-

- Calories: ~150
- Protein: ~5g
- Fiber: ~6g
- Cooking Time: 5 minutes

4. Chia Seed Pudding with Berries

-Ingredients:-
- 2 tablespoons chia seeds
- 1/2 cup almond milk
- Mixed berries (blueberries, raspberries)

-Preparation:-
1. Mix chia seeds with almond milk in a jar.
2. Refrigerate for at least 2 hours or overnight.
3. Top with mixed berries before serving.

-Nutritional Value:-
- Calories: ~180
- Protein: ~5g
- Fiber: ~8g
- Cooking Time: 2 hours (mostly refrigeration time)

5. Almond and Date Energy Balls

-Ingredients:-
- 1 cup almonds
- 1 cup pitted dates

- 1 tablespoon chia seeds
- Unsweetened shredded coconut for coating

-Preparation:-
1. In a food processor, blend almonds, dates, and chia seeds until a sticky mixture forms.
2. Roll into small balls and coat with shredded coconut.
3. Refrigerate for at least 30 minutes before serving.

-Nutritional Value:-
- Calories: ~150
- Protein: ~5g
- Fiber: ~4g
- Cooking Time: 15 minutes

These snack recipes are designed to be nutritious and supportive of liver health. Adjust portion sizes based on individual needs and consult with healthcare professionals for any necessary modifications.

Conclusion

Adopting a Fatty Liver & Cirrhosis Diet Cookbook can significantly contribute to maintaining liver health and overall well-being. The carefully curated recipes presented in this cookbook prioritize nutrient-dense, liver-friendly ingredients, offering a diverse and flavorful array of meals for breakfast, lunch, dinner, and snacks. From wholesome grains like quinoa to lean proteins such as grilled chicken and fatty fish rich in omega-3s, each recipe is crafted to provide essential nutrients while minimizing the intake of saturated fats and processed sugars.

These recipes are not merely a collection of delicious meals; they serve as a dietary roadmap, emphasizing the importance of balanced nutrition for individuals with Fatty Liver or Cirrhosis. The inclusion of colorful fruits, vegetables, and antioxidant-rich ingredients aims to support liver function and reduce inflammation.

As you embark on this culinary journey, remember that making positive changes to your diet is an empowering step towards better health. Consistency is key, and by incorporating these recipes into your daily routine, you are taking proactive measures to nurture your liver and promote overall wellness.

Motivation is the driving force behind sustained lifestyle changes. Picture the vitality and energy that comes with a healthier liver. Envision the increased quality of life and the potential for improved liver function. Embrace the idea that every meal is an opportunity to nurture and heal your body.

In the words of Hippocrates, "Let food be thy medicine and medicine be thy food." By adopting and adapting to this Fatty Liver & Cirrhosis Diet Cookbook, you are choosing a path of self-care, providing your body with the essential tools it needs to thrive. Your health is an investment, and this cookbook serves as your guide to a nourishing and fulfilling lifestyle. Start today, savor each nutritious bite, and embrace the journey towards a healthier, happier you. Your liver, and indeed your entire body, will thank you for it.

www.ingramcontent.com/pod-product-compliance
Lightning Source LLC
Chambersburg PA
CBHW070723260726
48660CB00007B/2700